Fitness Log

N. Rey | darebee.com

First Printing, 2021.
ISBN 13: 978-1-84481-168-7
ISBN 10: 1-84481-168-9

Published by New Line Books, London

Warning and Disclaimer
Although every precaution has been taken to verify the accuracy of the information contained herein, the
author and publisher assume no responsibility for any errors or omissions. No liability is assumed for
damage or injury that may result from the use of information contained within.

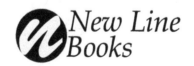

New Line
Books

About the Author

Neila Rey is the founder of Darebee, a global fitness resource. She is committed to democratizing fitness by removing the barriers to it and increasing accessibility. Every workout published in her books utilizes the latest in exercise science and has undergone thorough field testing and refinement through Darebee volunteers. When she's not busy running Darebee she is focused on finding fresh ways to make exercise easier and more enjoyable.

Introduction

If you can't measure something you can't track it. If you can't track it you can't affect it. If you can't affect it you can't improve it. These are all logical assumptions. The moment you apply them to fitness, wellbeing and nutrition they become part of the key requirements for building a better, future self.

There is a lot of scientific evidence that shows we can become healthier and can even improve on the way we feel when we consistently track specific habits and behaviors over a period of time. The reason we need to track specific aspects of our life that determine how healthy we become and how good we feel is that the world is complex and each day throws many complicated issues at us.

It's easy to get lost in the weeds. It's also equally easy to fall into the trap of tracking things for the sake of tracking and take away the accomplishment of having tracked them without any further benefit being derived from that activity.

Studies of patients with serious and potentially life-threatening conditions have found that even in such situations, unless there is a clear understanding of the reason the data is being tracked and the goals it will be sued for, tracking can become an end in itself.

Seek Meaning In Life As Well As Data

Exhaustive, detailed and compulsive data tracking that has no real goal beyond the tracking of the data in question is meaningless. The tracking of many complex parameters at once can also become meaningless very quickly. Fitness is an attribute that emerges from a fluid, biological environment where no two days or, indeed, no two moments are exactly the same.

We currently lack the analytics necessary to adequately track our everyday performance at every level possible and calculate it in a way that helps us make sense of the variables we keep track of. That doesn't mean however that we shouldn't try. As long as we keep track of specific, measurable variables which are key to our reaching specific goals we stand a really good chance of creating meaningful change in our health and fitness habits and behavior. By association, we also create meaningful change in our life.

The *100 Days of Change* is a fitness log that gets around a lot of the major issues associated with routine fitness tracking. It is relatively short in duration, yet long enough to allow physical and psychological effects to become apparent.

Because it is short it is seems like a reasonable length of time to devote to tracking specific elements of health and fitness. At the same time, because it is short, it allows for readjustment so what is being tracked can be improved and, once the tracking period is over, future goals can be also adjusted accordingly or we can better align our current behavior with what we want to attain in the future.

The parameters being tracked are few enough to not overwhelm us and sufficient in number and scope to cover our fitness and health progression needs, both inside and out. The guide makes us accountable to ourselves. By filling it in, over one hundred days, we take greater personal responsibility for our mental, physical and psychological improvement.

Our fitness journey then becomes more meaningful and more rewarding.

Date _____

Exercise Log

_____

_____

_____

_____

_____

_____

_____

_____

_____

_____

_____

_____

Muscles Worked

Total Time _____

Intensity   1   2   3   4   5

Mood   ☹ 😐 🙂 😃

Overall   ★ ★ ★ ★ ★

Food Log

_____

_____

_____

_____

_____

_____

_____

Liquids Log

_____

_____

_____

_____

_____

_____

_____

Sleep
total time _____

Meditation
total time _____

Notes

Date

Exercise Log

_____

_____

_____

_____

_____

_____

_____

_____

_____

_____

_____

_____

Muscles Worked

Total Time _____

Intensity   1   2   3   4   5

Mood   :(:| :)   :D

Overall   ★ ★ ★ ★ ★

Food Log

_____

_____

_____

_____

_____

_____

_____

Liquids Log

_____

_____

_____

_____

_____

_____

_____

Sleep total time _____

Meditation total time _____

Notes

Date _____

Exercise Log

_____
_____
_____
_____
_____
_____
_____
_____
_____
_____
_____
_____
_____

Muscles Worked

Total Time _____

Intensity   1   2   3   4   5

Mood   ☹   😐   🙂   😀

Overall   ★ ★ ★ ★ ★

Food Log

_____
_____
_____
_____
_____
_____

Liquids Log

_____
_____
_____
_____
_____
_____

Sleep
total time _____

Meditation
total time _____

Notes

Date _____

Exercise Log

_____

_____

_____

_____

_____

_____

_____

_____

_____

_____

_____

_____

Muscles Worked

Total Time _____

Intensity   1   2   3   4   5

Mood   :(:| :)   :D

Overall   ★ ★ ★ ★ ★

Food Log

_____

_____

_____

_____

_____

_____

_____

Liquids Log

_____

_____

_____

_____

_____

_____

_____

Sleep
total time _____

Meditation
total time _____

Notes

Date

Exercise Log

_____

_____

_____

_____

_____

_____

_____

_____

_____

_____

Muscles Worked

Total Time _____

Intensity   1   2   3   4   5

Mood   ☹   😐   🙂   😃

Overall   ★ ★ ★ ★ ★

Food Log

Liquids Log

_____

_____

_____

_____

_____

_____

_____

_____

_____

_____

_____

_____

_____

_____

Sleep
total time _____

Meditation
total time _____

Notes

Date

Exercise Log

_____

_____

_____

_____

_____

_____

_____

_____

_____

_____

_____

_____

Muscles Worked

Total Time _____

Intensity   1   2   3   4   5

Mood   ☹   😐   🙂   😃

Overall   ★ ★ ★ ★ ★

Food Log

_____

_____

_____

_____

_____

_____

_____

Liquids Log

_____

_____

_____

_____

_____

_____

_____

Sleep
total time _____

Meditation
total time _____

Notes

Date

Exercise Log

Muscles Worked

_____

_____

_____

_____

_____

_____

_____

_____

_____

_____

_____

_____

Total Time _____

Intensity   1   2   3   4   5

Mood   ☹   😐   🙂   😃

Overall   ★ ★ ★ ★ ★

Food Log

_____

_____

_____

_____

_____

_____

_____

_____

Liquids Log

_____

_____

_____

_____

_____

_____

_____

_____

Sleep
total time _____

Meditation
total time _____

Notes

Date

Exercise Log

_____

_____

_____

_____

_____

_____

_____

_____

_____

_____

_____

_____

Muscles Worked

Total Time _____

Intensity   1   2   3   4   5

Mood   ☹   😐   🙂   😃

Overall   ★ ★ ★ ★ ★

Food Log

_____

_____

_____

_____

_____

_____

Liquids Log

_____

_____

_____

_____

_____

_____

Sleep
total time _____

Meditation
total time _____

Notes

Date _____

Exercise Log

_____

_____

_____

_____

_____

_____

_____

_____

_____

_____

_____

Muscles Worked

Total Time _____

Intensity   1 2 3 4 5

Mood ☹ 😐 🙂 😀

Overall ★★★★★

Food Log

_____

_____

_____

_____

_____

_____

_____

Liquids Log

_____

_____

_____

_____

_____

_____

_____

Sleep
total time _____

Meditation
total time _____

Notes

Date _____

Exercise Log

_____

_____

_____

_____

_____

_____

_____

_____

_____

_____

_____

_____

Muscles Worked

Total Time _____

Intensity   1   2   3   4   5

Mood   ☹   😐   🙂   😀

Overall   ⭐ ⭐ ⭐ ⭐ ⭐

Food Log

_____
_____
_____
_____
_____
_____
_____

Liquids Log

_____
_____
_____
_____
_____
_____
_____

Sleep
total time _____

Meditation
total time _____

Notes

Date

Exercise Log

_____

_____

_____

_____

_____

_____

_____

_____

_____

_____

_____

_____

Muscles Worked

Total Time _____

Intensity 1 2 3 4 5

Mood ☹ 😐 🙂 😃

Overall ★ ★ ★ ★ ★

Food Log

_____

_____

_____

_____

_____

_____

_____

Liquids Log

_____

_____

_____

_____

_____

_____

_____

Sleep
total time _____

Meditation
total time _____

Notes

Date

Exercise Log

_____

_____

_____

_____

_____

_____

_____

_____

_____

_____

_____

Muscles Worked

Total Time _____

Intensity   1   2   3   4   5

Mood   ☹   😐   🙂   😃

Overall   ★ ★ ★ ★ ★

Food Log   Liquids Log

_____   _____

_____   _____

_____   _____

_____   _____

_____   _____

_____   _____

_____   _____

Sleep   Meditation
total time _____   total time _____

Notes

Date

Exercise Log

_____

_____

_____

_____

_____

_____

_____

_____

_____

_____

_____

_____

Muscles Worked

Total Time _____

Intensity   1 2 3 4 5

Mood   ☹ 😐 🙂 😃

Overall   ★ ★ ★ ★ ★

Food Log

_____

_____

_____

_____

_____

_____

_____

Liquids Log

_____

_____

_____

_____

_____

_____

_____

Sleep
total time _____

Meditation
total time _____

Notes

Date

Exercise Log

_____

_____

_____

_____

_____

_____

_____

_____

_____

_____

Muscles Worked

Total Time _____

Intensity   1   2   3   4   5

Mood   :(:| :)   :D

Overall   ★ ★ ★ ★ ★

Food Log

_____

_____

_____

_____

_____

_____

_____

_____

Liquids Log

_____

_____

_____

_____

_____

_____

_____

_____

Sleep
total time _____

Meditation
total time _____

Notes

Date _____

Exercise Log

_____

_____

_____

_____

_____

_____

_____

_____

_____

_____

_____

Muscles Worked

Total Time _____

Intensity   1   2   3   4   5

Mood   ☹   😐   🙂   😀

Overall   ★ ★ ★ ★ ★

Food Log

_____

_____

_____

_____

_____

_____

_____

Liquids Log

_____

_____

_____

_____

_____

_____

_____

Sleep
total time _____

Meditation
total time _____

Notes

Date

Exercise Log

Muscles Worked

Total Time _____

Intensity   1   2   3   4   5

Mood   ☹   😐   🙂   😃

Overall ⭐⭐⭐⭐⭐

Food Log

_____

_____

_____

_____

_____

_____

_____

Liquids Log

_____

_____

_____

_____

_____

_____

_____

Sleep
total time _____

Meditation
total time _____

Notes

Date

Exercise Log

_____

_____

_____

_____

_____

_____

_____

_____

_____

_____

_____

_____

Muscles Worked

Total Time _____

Intensity   1   2   3   4   5

Mood   ☹   😐   🙂   😃

Overall   ★ ★ ★ ★ ★

Food Log

_____

_____

_____

_____

_____

_____

_____

Liquids Log

_____

_____

_____

_____

_____

_____

_____

Sleep
total time _____

Meditation
total time _____

Notes

Date

Exercise Log

_____

_____

_____

_____

_____

_____

_____

_____

_____

_____

_____

Muscles Worked

Total Time _____

Intensity   1   2   3   4   5

Mood   🙁   😐   🙂   😃

Overall ⭐ ⭐ ⭐ ⭐ ⭐

Food Log

_____

_____

_____

_____

_____

_____

_____

Liquids Log

_____

_____

_____

_____

_____

_____

_____

Sleep
total time _____

Meditation
total time _____

Notes

Date

Exercise Log

_____

_____

_____

_____

_____

_____

_____

_____

_____

_____

_____

Muscles Worked

Total Time _____

Intensity   1   2   3   4   5

Mood   ☹   😐   🙂   😃

Overall   ★ ★ ★ ★ ★

Food Log

_____

_____

_____

_____

_____

_____

_____

Liquids Log

_____

_____

_____

_____

_____

_____

_____

Sleep
total time _____

Meditation
total time _____

Notes

Date

Exercise Log

_____

_____

_____

_____

_____

_____

_____

_____

_____

_____

_____

_____

_____

_____

Muscles Worked

Total Time _____

Intensity   1   2   3   4   5

Mood   :(:| :)   :D

Overall   ★ ★ ★ ★ ★

Food Log

Liquids Log

_____

_____

_____

_____

_____

_____

_____

_____

_____

_____

_____

_____

_____

_____

Sleep
total time _____

Meditation
total time _____

Notes

Date _____

Exercise Log

_____

_____

_____

_____

_____

_____

_____

_____

_____

_____

_____

_____

Muscles Worked

Total Time _____

Intensity   1   2   3   4   5

Mood   ☹   😐   🙂   😀

Overall   ★ ★ ★ ★ ★

Food Log

_____

_____

_____

_____

_____

_____

_____

Liquids Log

_____

_____

_____

_____

_____

_____

_____

Sleep
total time _____

Meditation
total time _____

Notes

Date

Exercise Log

_____

_____

_____

_____

_____

_____

_____

_____

_____

_____

_____

Muscles Worked

Total Time _____

Intensity   1   2   3   4   5

Mood   ☹   😐   🙂   😃

Overall   ★ ★ ★ ★ ★

Food Log

_____

_____

_____

_____

_____

_____

_____

Liquids Log

_____

_____

_____

_____

_____

_____

_____

Sleep
total time _____

Meditation
total time _____

Notes

Date _____

Exercise Log

_____

_____

_____

_____

_____

_____

_____

_____

_____

_____

_____

_____

Muscles Worked

Total Time _____

Intensity   1   2   3   4   5

Mood   ☹   😐   🙂   😃

Overall   ★ ★ ★ ★ ★

Food Log

_____

_____

_____

_____

_____

_____

_____

Liquids Log

_____

_____

_____

_____

_____

_____

_____

Sleep
total time _____

Meditation
total time _____

Notes

Date _____

Exercise Log

_____

_____

_____

_____

_____

_____

_____

_____

_____

_____

_____

Muscles Worked

Total Time _____

Intensity   1   2   3   4   5

Mood   ☹   😐   🙂   😃

Overall   ★ ★ ★ ★ ★

Food Log

_____

_____

_____

_____

_____

_____

_____

Liquids Log

_____

_____

_____

_____

_____

_____

_____

Sleep
total time _____

Meditation
total time _____

Notes

Date _____

Exercise Log

_____

_____

_____

_____

_____

_____

_____

_____

_____

_____

_____

_____

_____

Muscles Worked

Total Time _____

Intensity   1   2   3   4   5

Mood   ☹   😐   🙂   😃

Overall   ★ ★ ★ ★ ★

Food Log

_____

_____

_____

_____

_____

_____

_____

Liquids Log

_____

_____

_____

_____

_____

_____

_____

Sleep
total time _____

Meditation
total time _____

Notes

Date _____

Exercise Log

_____

_____

_____

_____

_____

_____

_____

_____

_____

_____

_____

_____

Muscles Worked

Total Time _____

Intensity   1   2   3   4   5

Mood   ☹   😐   🙂   😃

Overall   ★ ★ ★ ★ ★

Food Log

_____

_____

_____

_____

_____

_____

_____

Liquids Log

_____

_____

_____

_____

_____

_____

_____

Sleep
total time _____

Meditation
total time _____

Notes

Date _____

Exercise Log

_____
_____
_____
_____
_____
_____
_____
_____
_____
_____
_____
_____
_____

Muscles Worked

Total Time _____

Intensity   1   2   3   4   5

Mood   ☹   😐   🙂   😃

Overall   ★ ★ ★ ★ ★

Food Log

_____

_____

_____

_____

_____

_____

_____

Liquids Log

_____

_____

_____

_____

_____

_____

_____

Sleep
total time _____

Meditation
total time _____

Notes

Date

Exercise Log

_____

_____

_____

_____

_____

_____

_____

_____

_____

_____

_____

_____

Muscles Worked

Total Time _____

Intensity   1   2   3   4   5

Mood   ☹   😐   🙂   😃

Overall   ★ ★ ★ ★ ★

Food Log

_____

_____

_____

_____

_____

_____

_____

Liquids Log

_____

_____

_____

_____

_____

_____

_____

Sleep
total time _____

Meditation
total time _____

Notes

Date _____

Exercise Log

_____

_____

_____

_____

_____

_____

_____

_____

_____

_____

_____

_____

Muscles Worked

Total Time _____

Intensity   1   2   3   4   5

Mood   ☹   😐   🙂   😀

Overall   ★ ★ ★ ★ ★

Food Log

_____

_____

_____

_____

_____

_____

_____

Liquids Log

_____

_____

_____

_____

_____

_____

_____

Sleep
total time _____

Meditation
total time _____

Notes

Date _____

Exercise Log

_____

_____

_____

_____

_____

_____

_____

_____

_____

_____

_____

Muscles Worked

Total Time _____

Intensity 1 2 3 4 5

Mood ☹ 😐 🙂 😃

Overall ★ ★ ★ ★ ★

Food Log

_____

_____

_____

_____

_____

_____

_____

Liquids Log

_____

_____

_____

_____

_____

_____

_____

Sleep
total time _____

Meditation
total time _____

Notes

Date _____

Exercise Log

_____
_____
_____
_____
_____
_____
_____
_____
_____
_____
_____
_____

Muscles Worked

Total Time _____

Intensity   1 2 3 4 5

Mood   ☹ 😐 🙂 😃

Overall   ★★★★★

Food Log

_____

_____

_____

_____

_____

_____

_____

Liquids Log

_____

_____

_____

_____

_____

_____

_____

Sleep
total time _____

Meditation
total time _____

Notes

Date _____

Exercise Log

_____

_____

_____

_____

_____

_____

_____

_____

_____

_____

_____

_____

Muscles Worked

Total Time _____

Intensity   1   2   3   4   5

Mood   ☹   😐   🙂   😃

Overall   ⭐ ⭐ ⭐ ⭐ ⭐

Food Log

_____

_____

_____

_____

_____

_____

_____

Liquids Log

_____

_____

_____

_____

_____

_____

_____

Sleep
total time _____

Meditation
total time _____

Notes

Date _____

Exercise Log

_____

_____

_____

_____

_____

_____

_____

_____

_____

_____

_____

_____

_____

_____

Muscles Worked

Total Time _____

Intensity   1   2   3   4   5

Mood   ☹   😐   🙂   😃

Overall   ★ ★ ★ ★ ★

Food Log

_____

_____

_____

_____

_____

_____

Liquids Log

_____

_____

_____

_____

_____

_____

Sleep
total time _____

Meditation
total time _____

Notes

Date

Exercise Log

_____

_____

_____

_____

_____

_____

_____

_____

_____

_____

_____

_____

Muscles Worked

Total Time _____

Intensity 1 2 3 4 5

Mood ☹ 😐 🙂 😀

Overall ★★★★★

Food Log

_____
_____
_____
_____
_____
_____
_____

Liquids Log

_____
_____
_____
_____
_____
_____
_____

Sleep
total time _____

Meditation
total time _____

Notes

Date _____

Exercise Log

_____
_____
_____
_____
_____
_____
_____
_____
_____
_____
_____
_____

Muscles Worked

Total Time _____

Intensity   1   2   3   4   5

Mood   ☹   😐   🙂   😃

Overall   ★ ★ ★ ★ ★

Food Log

_____

_____

_____

_____

_____

_____

_____

Liquids Log

_____

_____

_____

_____

_____

_____

_____

Sleep
total time _____

Meditation
total time _____

Notes

Date _____

Exercise Log

_____

_____

_____

_____

_____

_____

_____

_____

_____

_____

_____

_____

Muscles Worked

Total Time _____

Intensity   1 2 3 4 5

Mood   ☹ 😐 🙂 😃

Overall ⭐ ⭐ ⭐ ⭐ ⭐

Food Log

_____

_____

_____

_____

_____

_____

_____

_____

Liquids Log

_____

_____

_____

_____

_____

_____

_____

_____

Sleep
total time _____

Meditation
total time _____

Notes

Date _____

Exercise Log

_____

_____

_____

_____

_____

_____

_____

_____

_____

_____

_____

_____

Muscles Worked

Total Time _____

Intensity   1   2   3   4   5

Mood   :(:| :)   :D

Overall   ★ ★ ★ ★ ★

Food Log

_____

_____

_____

_____

_____

_____

_____

Liquids Log

_____

_____

_____

_____

_____

_____

_____

Sleep
total time _____

Meditation
total time _____

Notes

Date

Exercise Log

_____

_____

_____

_____

_____

_____

_____

_____

_____

_____

_____

Muscles Worked

Total Time _____

Intensity   1   2   3   4   5

Mood   :(:| :)   :D

Overall   ★ ★ ★ ★ ★

Food Log

_____

_____

_____

_____

_____

_____

_____

Liquids Log

_____

_____

_____

_____

_____

_____

_____

Sleep
total time _____

Meditation
total time _____

Notes

Date _____

Exercise Log

_____

_____

_____

_____

_____

_____

_____

_____

_____

_____

_____

Muscles Worked

Total Time _____

Intensity   1   2   3   4   5

Mood   :(:| :)   :D

Overall   ★ ★ ★ ★ ★

Food Log

_____
_____
_____
_____
_____
_____
_____

Liquids Log

_____
_____
_____
_____
_____
_____
_____

Sleep
total time _____

Meditation
total time _____

Notes

Date

Exercise Log

_____

_____

_____

_____

_____

_____

_____

_____

_____

_____

_____

_____

Muscles Worked

Total Time _____

Intensity 1 2 3 4 5

Mood ☹ 😐 🙂 😀

Overall ★★★★★

Food Log

_____

_____

_____

_____

_____

_____

_____

_____

Liquids Log

_____

_____

_____

_____

_____

_____

_____

_____

Sleep
total time _____

Meditation
total time _____

Notes

Date _____

Exercise Log

_____

_____

_____

_____

_____

_____

_____

_____

_____

_____

_____

_____

Muscles Worked

Total Time _____

Intensity   1   2   3   4   5

Mood   :(:| :)   :D

Overall   ★ ★ ★ ★ ★

Food Log

_____

_____

_____

_____

_____

_____

_____

Liquids Log

_____

_____

_____

_____

_____

_____

_____

Sleep
total time _____

Meditation
total time _____

Notes

Date _____

Exercise Log

_____
_____
_____
_____
_____
_____
_____
_____
_____
_____
_____

Muscles Worked

Total Time _____

Intensity   1   2   3   4   5

Mood   ☹   😐   🙂   😀

Overall   ⭐ ⭐ ⭐ ⭐ ⭐

Food Log

_____

_____

_____

_____

_____

_____

_____

_____

Liquids Log

_____

_____

_____

_____

_____

_____

_____

_____

Sleep
total time _____

Meditation
total time _____

Notes

Date

Exercise Log

_____

_____

_____

_____

_____

_____

_____

_____

_____

_____

_____

_____

Muscles Worked

Total Time _____

Intensity   1   2   3   4   5

Mood   :(:| :)   :D

Overall   ★ ★ ★ ★ ★

Food Log

_____

_____

_____

_____

_____

_____

_____

Liquids Log

_____

_____

_____

_____

_____

_____

_____

Sleep
total time _____

Meditation
total time _____

Notes

Date

Exercise Log

Muscles Worked

_____

_____

_____

_____

_____

_____

_____

_____

_____

_____

_____

_____

_____

Total Time

_____

Intensity   1 2 3 4 5

Mood   :(:| :)   :D

Overall   ★★★★★

Food Log

_____

_____

_____

_____

_____

_____

_____

Liquids Log

_____

_____

_____

_____

_____

_____

_____

Sleep
total time _____

Meditation
total time _____

Notes

Date

Exercise Log

_____

_____

_____

_____

_____

_____

_____

_____

_____

_____

_____

Muscles Worked

Total Time _____

Intensity   1 2 3 4 5

Mood   ☹ ☺ ☺ ☺

Overall   ★★★★★

Food Log

_____

_____

_____

_____

_____

_____

_____

Liquids Log

_____

_____

_____

_____

_____

_____

_____

Sleep
total time _____

Meditation
total time _____

Notes

Date

Exercise Log

_____

_____

_____

_____

_____

_____

_____

_____

_____

_____

_____

Muscles Worked

Total Time _____

Intensity   1 2 3 4 5

Mood   ☹ 😐 🙂 😄

Overall   ★★★★★

Food Log

Liquids Log

Sleep
total time _____

Meditation
total time _____

Notes

Date _____

Exercise Log

_____

_____

_____

_____

_____

_____

_____

_____

_____

_____

_____

_____

Muscles Worked

Total Time _____

Intensity   1 2 3 4 5

Mood   :(:| :)   :D

Overall   ★ ★ ★ ★ ★

Food Log

_____

_____

_____

_____

_____

_____

_____

Liquids Log

_____

_____

_____

_____

_____

_____

_____

Sleep
total time _____

Meditation
total time _____

Notes

Date _____

Exercise Log

_____

_____

_____

_____

_____

_____

_____

_____

_____

_____

_____

Muscles Worked

Total Time _____

Intensity   1   2   3   4   5

Mood   ☹   😐   🙂   😃

Overall   ★ ★ ★ ★ ★

Food Log   Liquids Log

_____   _____

_____   _____

_____   _____

_____   _____

_____   _____

_____   _____

_____   _____

_____   _____

Sleep   Meditation
total time _____   total time _____

————————————————— Notes —————————————————

```



```

Date _____

Exercise Log

_____

_____

_____

_____

_____

_____

_____

_____

_____

_____

_____

Muscles Worked

Total Time _____

Intensity   1   2   3   4   5

Mood   ☹   😐   🙂   😃

Overall   ★ ★ ★ ★ ★

Food Log

_____

_____

_____

_____

_____

_____

_____

_____

Liquids Log

_____

_____

_____

_____

_____

_____

_____

_____

Sleep
total time _____

Meditation
total time _____

Notes

Date

Exercise Log

Muscles Worked

_____

_____

_____

_____

_____

_____

_____

_____

_____

_____

_____

Total Time _____

Intensity   1   2   3   4   5

Mood   ☹   😐   🙂   😀

Overall   ★ ★ ★ ★ ★

Food Log

_____

_____

_____

_____

_____

_____

_____

Liquids Log

_____

_____

_____

_____

_____

_____

_____

Sleep
total time _____

Meditation
total time _____

Notes

Date _____

Exercise Log

_____

_____

_____

_____

_____

_____

_____

_____

_____

_____

_____

_____

Muscles Worked

Total Time _____

Intensity   1   2   3   4   5

Mood   ☹   😐   🙂   😀

Overall   ★ ★ ★ ★ ★

Food Log

_____

_____

_____

_____

_____

_____

_____

Liquids Log

_____

_____

_____

_____

_____

_____

_____

Sleep
total time _____

Meditation
total time _____

Notes

Date

Exercise Log

_____

_____

_____

_____

_____

_____

_____

_____

_____

_____

_____

Muscles Worked

Total Time _____

Intensity   1   2   3   4   5

Mood   :(:| :)   :D

Overall   ★ ★ ★ ★ ★

Food Log

_____

_____

_____

_____

_____

_____

_____

Liquids Log

_____

_____

_____

_____

_____

_____

_____

Sleep
total time _____

Meditation
total time _____

Notes

Date

Exercise Log

_____

_____

_____

_____

_____

_____

_____

_____

_____

_____

_____

Muscles Worked

Total Time _____

Intensity   1   2   3   4   5

Mood   ☹   😐   🙂   😄

Overall   ★ ★ ★ ★ ★

Food Log

_____

_____

_____

_____

_____

_____

_____

Liquids Log

_____

_____

_____

_____

_____

_____

_____

Sleep
total time _____

Meditation
total time _____

Notes

Date _____

Exercise Log

_____

_____

_____

_____

_____

_____

_____

_____

_____

_____

_____

Muscles Worked

Total Time _____

Intensity   1   2   3   4   5

Mood   ☹   😐   🙂   😃

Overall   ⭐ ⭐ ⭐ ⭐ ⭐

Food Log

_____
_____
_____
_____
_____
_____
_____
_____

Liquids Log

_____
_____
_____
_____
_____
_____
_____
_____

Sleep
total time _____

Meditation
total time _____

Notes

Date

Exercise Log

_____

_____

_____

_____

_____

_____

_____

_____

_____

_____

_____

_____

Muscles Worked

Total Time _____

Intensity 1 2 3 4 5

Mood ☹ 😐 🙂 😃

Overall ★ ★ ★ ★ ★

Food Log

_____

_____

_____

_____

_____

_____

_____

Liquids Log

_____

_____

_____

_____

_____

_____

_____

Sleep
total time _____

Meditation
total time _____

Notes

Date _____

Exercise Log

_____

_____

_____

_____

_____

_____

_____

_____

_____

_____

_____

Muscles Worked

Total Time _____

Intensity   1   2   3   4   5

Mood   ☹   😐   🙂   😃

Overall   ★ ★ ★ ★ ★

Food Log

_____

_____

_____

_____

_____

_____

_____

Liquids Log

_____

_____

_____

_____

_____

_____

_____

Sleep
total time _____

Meditation
total time _____

Notes

Date

Exercise Log

_____

_____

_____

_____

_____

_____

_____

_____

_____

_____

_____

_____

Muscles Worked

Total Time _____

Intensity   1   2   3   4   5

Mood   ☹   😐   🙂   😃

Overall   ★ ★ ★ ★ ★

Food Log

_____

_____

_____

_____

_____

_____

_____

Liquids Log

_____

_____

_____

_____

_____

_____

_____

Sleep
total time _____

Meditation
total time _____

Notes

Date _____

Exercise Log

_____

_____

_____

_____

_____

_____

_____

_____

_____

_____

_____

Muscles Worked

Total Time _____

Intensity   1   2   3   4   5

Mood   :(:| :)   :D

Overall   ★ ★ ★ ★ ★

Food Log

_____
_____
_____
_____
_____
_____
_____
_____
_____

Liquids Log

_____
_____
_____
_____
_____
_____
_____
_____
_____

Sleep
total time _____

Meditation
total time _____

Notes

Date

Exercise Log

_____

_____

_____

_____

_____

_____

_____

_____

_____

_____

_____

_____

Muscles Worked

Total Time _____

Intensity   1   2   3   4   5

Mood   :(:| :)   :D

Overall   ★ ★ ★ ★ ★

Food Log

_____

_____

_____

_____

_____

_____

_____

Liquids Log

_____

_____

_____

_____

_____

_____

_____

Sleep
total time _____

Meditation
total time _____

Notes

Date _____

Exercise Log

_____

_____

_____

_____

_____

_____

_____

_____

_____

_____

Muscles Worked

Total Time _____

Intensity   1   2   3   4   5

Mood   :(:| :)   :D

Overall   ★ ★ ★ ★ ★

Food Log

_____

_____

_____

_____

_____

_____

_____

Liquids Log

_____

_____

_____

_____

_____

_____

_____

Sleep total time _____

Meditation total time _____

Notes

Date

Exercise Log

_____

_____

_____

_____

_____

_____

_____

_____

_____

_____

_____

Muscles Worked

Total Time _____

Intensity   1   2   3   4   5

Mood   ☹   😐   🙂   😀

Overall   ★ ★ ★ ★ ★

Food Log

_____

_____

_____

_____

_____

_____

_____

Liquids Log

_____

_____

_____

_____

_____

_____

_____

Sleep
total time _____

Meditation
total time _____

Notes

Date _____

Exercise Log

_____

_____

_____

_____

_____

_____

_____

_____

_____

_____

_____

_____

Muscles Worked

Total Time _____

Intensity   1   2   3   4   5

Mood   ☹   😐   🙂   😃

Overall   ★ ★ ★ ★ ★

Food Log

_____

_____

_____

_____

_____

_____

_____

Liquids Log

_____

_____

_____

_____

_____

_____

_____

Sleep
total time _____

Meditation
total time _____

Notes

Date _____

Exercise Log

_____
_____
_____
_____
_____
_____
_____
_____
_____
_____
_____
_____

Muscles Worked

Total Time _____

Intensity   1 2 3 4 5

Mood   ☹ 😐 🙂 😀

Overall   ★ ★ ★ ★ ★

Food Log

_____

_____

_____

_____

_____

_____

_____

Liquids Log

_____

_____

_____

_____

_____

_____

_____

Sleep
total time _____

Meditation
total time _____

Notes

Date

Exercise Log

_____

_____

_____

_____

_____

_____

_____

_____

_____

_____

_____

Muscles Worked

Total Time _____

Intensity   1   2   3   4   5

Mood   ☹   😐   🙂   😄

Overall   ★ ★ ★ ★ ★

Food Log

_____

_____

_____

_____

_____

_____

_____

Liquids Log

_____

_____

_____

_____

_____

_____

_____

Sleep
total time _____

Meditation
total time _____

Notes

Date _____

Exercise Log

_____

_____

_____

_____

_____

_____

_____

_____

_____

_____

_____

Muscles Worked

Total Time _____

Intensity   1   2   3   4   5

Mood   ☹   😐   🙂   😃

Overall   ★ ★ ★ ★ ★

Food Log

_____

_____

_____

_____

_____

_____

_____

_____

Liquids Log

_____

_____

_____

_____

_____

_____

_____

_____

Sleep
total time _____

Meditation
total time _____

Notes

Date

Exercise Log

_____

_____

_____

_____

_____

_____

_____

_____

_____

_____

_____

Muscles Worked

Total Time _____

Intensity   1   2   3   4   5

Mood   ☹   😐   🙂   😃

Overall   ★ ★ ★ ★ ★

Food Log

_____

_____

_____

_____

_____

_____

_____

Liquids Log

_____

_____

_____

_____

_____

_____

_____

Sleep
total time _____

Meditation
total time _____

Notes

Date

Exercise Log

_____

_____

_____

_____

_____

_____

_____

_____

_____

_____

_____

_____

Muscles Worked

Total Time _____

Intensity   1   2   3   4   5

Mood   ☹   😐   🙂   😃

Overall   ★ ★ ★ ★ ★

Food Log

_____

_____

_____

_____

_____

_____

Liquids Log

_____

_____

_____

_____

_____

_____

Sleep
total time _____

Meditation
total time _____

Notes

Date

Exercise Log

_____

_____

_____

_____

_____

_____

_____

_____

_____

_____

_____

Muscles Worked

Total Time _____

Intensity   1   2   3   4   5

Mood   ☹   😐   🙂   😃

Overall   ★ ★ ★ ★ ★

Food Log

_____

_____

_____

_____

_____

_____

_____

Liquids Log

_____

_____

_____

_____

_____

_____

_____

Sleep
total time _____

Meditation
total time _____

Notes

Date

Exercise Log

_____

_____

_____

_____

_____

_____

_____

_____

_____

_____

_____

_____

Muscles Worked

Total Time _____

Intensity   1   2   3   4   5

Mood   ☹   😐   🙂   😀

Overall   ★ ★ ★ ★ ★

Food Log

_____

_____

_____

_____

_____

_____

_____

_____

Liquids Log

_____

_____

_____

_____

_____

_____

_____

_____

Sleep
total time _____

Meditation
total time _____

Notes

Date

Exercise Log

_____

_____

_____

_____

_____

_____

_____

_____

_____

_____

_____

_____

Muscles Worked

Total Time _____

Intensity   1   2   3   4   5

Mood   ☹   😐   🙂   😃

Overall   ★ ★ ★ ★ ★

Food Log

_____

_____

_____

_____

_____

_____

_____

Liquids Log

_____

_____

_____

_____

_____

_____

_____

Sleep
total time _____

Meditation
total time _____

Notes

Date _____

Exercise Log

_____

_____

_____

_____

_____

_____

_____

_____

_____

_____

_____

_____

Muscles Worked

Total Time _____

Intensity   1   2   3   4   5

Mood   :(:| :)   :D

Overall   ★ ★ ★ ★ ★

Food Log

_____

_____

_____

_____

_____

_____

_____

Liquids Log

_____

_____

_____

_____

_____

_____

_____

Sleep
total time _____

Meditation
total time _____

Notes

Date

Exercise Log

_____

_____

_____

_____

_____

_____

_____

_____

_____

_____

_____

_____

Muscles Worked

Total Time _____

Intensity   1   2   3   4   5

Mood   ☹   😐   🙂   😀

Overall   ★ ★ ★ ★ ★

Food Log

_____

_____

_____

_____

_____

_____

_____

Liquids Log

_____

_____

_____

_____

_____

_____

_____

Sleep
total time _____

Meditation
total time _____

Notes

Date _____

Exercise Log

_____
_____
_____
_____
_____
_____
_____
_____
_____
_____
_____
_____

Muscles Worked

Total Time _____

Intensity   1 2 3 4 5

Mood   ☹ 😐 🙂 😃

Overall   ★ ★ ★ ★ ★

Food Log

_____

_____

_____

_____

_____

_____

_____

Liquids Log

_____

_____

_____

_____

_____

_____

_____

Sleep
total time _____

Meditation
total time _____

Notes

Date

Exercise Log

_____

_____

_____

_____

_____

_____

_____

_____

_____

_____

_____

_____

Muscles Worked

Total Time _____

Intensity   1   2   3   4   5

Mood   ☹   😐   🙂   😀

Overall   ★ ★ ★ ★ ★

Food Log

_____

_____

_____

_____

_____

_____

_____

Liquids Log

_____

_____

_____

_____

_____

_____

_____

Sleep
total time _____

Meditation
total time _____

Notes

Date

Exercise Log

_____

_____

_____

_____

_____

_____

_____

_____

_____

_____

_____

Muscles Worked

Total Time

_____

Intensity   1   2   3   4   5

Mood   ☹   😐   🙂   😃

Overall   ★ ★ ★ ★ ★

Food Log

_____

_____

_____

_____

_____

_____

_____

Liquids Log

_____

_____

_____

_____

_____

_____

_____

Sleep
total time _____

Meditation
total time _____

Notes

Date _____

Exercise Log

_____

_____

_____

_____

_____

_____

_____

_____

_____

_____

_____

_____

Muscles Worked

Total Time _____

Intensity   1 2 3 4 5

Mood   ☹ 😐 🙂 😄

Overall ★ ★ ★ ★ ★

Food Log

_____

_____

_____

_____

_____

_____

_____

Liquids Log

_____

_____

_____

_____

_____

_____

_____

Sleep
total time _____

Meditation
total time _____

Notes

Date _____

Exercise Log

_____

_____

_____

_____

_____

_____

_____

_____

_____

_____

_____

_____

Muscles Worked

Total Time _____

Intensity   1   2   3   4   5

Mood   ☹   😐   🙂   😄

Overall   ★ ★ ★ ★ ★

Food Log

_____

_____

_____

_____

_____

_____

_____

_____

Liquids Log

_____

_____

_____

_____

_____

_____

_____

_____

Sleep
total time _____

Meditation
total time _____

Notes

Date _____

Exercise Log

_____

_____

_____

_____

_____

_____

_____

_____

_____

_____

_____

Muscles Worked

Total Time _____

Intensity   1   2   3   4   5

Mood   :(:| :)   :D

Overall   ★ ★ ★ ★ ★

Food Log

_____

_____

_____

_____

_____

_____

_____

_____

Liquids Log

_____

_____

_____

_____

_____

_____

_____

_____

Sleep
total time _____

Meditation
total time _____

Notes

Date _____

Exercise Log

_____

_____

_____

_____

_____

_____

_____

_____

_____

_____

_____

_____

Muscles Worked

Total Time _____

Intensity   1   2   3   4   5

Mood   ☹   😐   🙂   😃

Overall   ★ ★ ★ ★ ★

Food Log

_____

_____

_____

_____

_____

_____

_____

Liquids Log

_____

_____

_____

_____

_____

_____

_____

Sleep
total time _____

Meditation
total time _____

Notes

Date _____

Exercise Log

_____

_____

_____

_____

_____

_____

_____

_____

_____

_____

_____

Muscles Worked

Total Time _____

Intensity   1   2   3   4   5

Mood   ☹   😐   🙂   😃

Overall   ⭐ ⭐ ⭐ ⭐ ⭐

Food Log

_____

_____

_____

_____

_____

_____

_____

Liquids Log

_____

_____

_____

_____

_____

_____

_____

Sleep
total time _____

Meditation
total time _____

Notes

Date _____

Exercise Log

_____

_____

_____

_____

_____

_____

_____

_____

_____

_____

_____

_____

Muscles Worked

Total Time _____

Intensity   1   2   3   4   5

Mood   ☹ 😐 🙂 😃

Overall   ★ ★ ★ ★ ★

Food Log

_____

_____

_____

_____

_____

_____

_____

Liquids Log

_____

_____

_____

_____

_____

_____

_____

Sleep
total time _____

Meditation
total time _____

Notes

Date

Exercise Log

_____

_____

_____

_____

_____

_____

_____

_____

_____

_____

Muscles Worked

Total Time _____

Intensity   1   2   3   4   5

Mood   ☹   😐   🙂   😃

Overall   ★ ★ ★ ★ ★

Food Log

_____

_____

_____

_____

_____

_____

_____

_____

Liquids Log

_____

_____

_____

_____

_____

_____

_____

_____

Sleep
total time _____

Meditation
total time _____

Notes

Date ⎯⎯⎯⎯⎯⎯⎯⎯⎯⎯

Exercise Log

⎯⎯⎯⎯⎯⎯⎯⎯⎯⎯⎯⎯⎯⎯⎯⎯

⎯⎯⎯⎯⎯⎯⎯⎯⎯⎯⎯⎯⎯⎯⎯⎯

⎯⎯⎯⎯⎯⎯⎯⎯⎯⎯⎯⎯⎯⎯⎯⎯

⎯⎯⎯⎯⎯⎯⎯⎯⎯⎯⎯⎯⎯⎯⎯⎯

⎯⎯⎯⎯⎯⎯⎯⎯⎯⎯⎯⎯⎯⎯⎯⎯

⎯⎯⎯⎯⎯⎯⎯⎯⎯⎯⎯⎯⎯⎯⎯⎯

⎯⎯⎯⎯⎯⎯⎯⎯⎯⎯⎯⎯⎯⎯⎯⎯

⎯⎯⎯⎯⎯⎯⎯⎯⎯⎯⎯⎯⎯⎯⎯⎯

⎯⎯⎯⎯⎯⎯⎯⎯⎯⎯⎯⎯⎯⎯⎯⎯

⎯⎯⎯⎯⎯⎯⎯⎯⎯⎯⎯⎯⎯⎯⎯⎯

Muscles Worked

Total Time ⎯⎯⎯⎯⎯⎯⎯⎯⎯

Intensity   1 2 3 4 5

Mood   ☹ 😐 🙂 😃

Overall   ★ ★ ★ ★ ★

Food Log

_____

_____

_____

_____

_____

_____

_____

Liquids Log

_____

_____

_____

_____

_____

_____

_____

Sleep
total time _____

Meditation
total time _____

Notes

Date _____

Exercise Log

_____

_____

_____

_____

_____

_____

_____

_____

_____

_____

_____

Muscles Worked

Total Time _____

Intensity 1 2 3 4 5

Mood ☹ 😐 🙂 😃

Overall ⭐ ⭐ ⭐ ⭐ ⭐

Food Log

_____

_____

_____

_____

_____

_____

_____

_____

Liquids Log

_____

_____

_____

_____

_____

_____

_____

_____

Sleep
total time _____

Meditation
total time _____

Notes

Date _____

Exercise Log

_____

_____

_____

_____

_____

_____

_____

_____

_____

_____

_____

Muscles Worked

Total Time _____

Intensity 1 2 3 4 5

Mood :(:| :) :D

Overall ★ ★ ★ ★ ★

Food Log

Liquids Log

_____

_____

_____

_____

_____

_____

_____

Sleep
total time _____

Meditation
total time _____

Notes

Date _____

Exercise Log

_____

_____

_____

_____

_____

_____

_____

_____

_____

_____

_____

Muscles Worked

Total Time _____

Intensity   1   2   3   4   5

Mood   ☹   😐   🙂   😃

Overall   ⭐ ⭐ ⭐ ⭐ ⭐

Food Log

_____

_____

_____

_____

_____

_____

_____

_____

Liquids Log

_____

_____

_____

_____

_____

_____

_____

_____

Sleep
total time _____

Meditation
total time _____

Notes

Date _____

Exercise Log

_____

_____

_____

_____

_____

_____

_____

_____

_____

_____

_____

Muscles Worked

Total Time _____

Intensity 1 2 3 4 5

Mood ☹ 😐 🙂 😄

Overall ★ ★ ★ ★ ★

Food Log

_____

_____

_____

_____

_____

_____

_____

Liquids Log

_____

_____

_____

_____

_____

_____

_____

Sleep
total time _____

Meditation
total time _____

Notes

Date

Exercise Log

_____

_____

_____

_____

_____

_____

_____

_____

_____

_____

Muscles Worked

Total Time _____

Intensity   1   2   3   4   5

Mood   ☹   😐   🙂   😃

Overall   ★ ★ ★ ★ ★

Food Log

_____

_____

_____

_____

_____

_____

_____

Liquids Log

_____

_____

_____

_____

_____

_____

_____

**Sleep
total time** _____

**Meditation
total time** _____

Notes

Date _____

Exercise Log

_____

_____

_____

_____

_____

_____

_____

_____

_____

_____

_____

_____

Muscles Worked

Total Time _____

Intensity   1   2   3   4   5

Mood   ☹   😐   🙂   😃

Overall   ⭐ ⭐ ⭐ ⭐ ⭐

Food Log

_____

_____

_____

_____

_____

_____

_____

Liquids Log

_____

_____

_____

_____

_____

_____

_____

Sleep
total time _____

Meditation
total time _____

Notes

Date _____

Exercise Log

_____

_____

_____

_____

_____

_____

_____

_____

_____

_____

_____

_____

Muscles Worked

Total Time _____

Intensity   1 2 3 4 5

Mood   ☹ 😐 🙂 😀

Overall ★★★★★

Food Log

_____

_____

_____

_____

_____

_____

_____

_____

Liquids Log

_____

_____

_____

_____

_____

_____

_____

_____

**Sleep
total time** _____

**Meditation
total time** _____

Notes

Date _____

Exercise Log

_____

_____

_____

_____

_____

_____

_____

_____

_____

_____

_____

_____

_____

Muscles Worked

Total Time _____

Intensity   1   2   3   4   5

Mood   ☹   😐   🙂   😃

Overall   ★ ★ ★ ★ ★

Food Log

_____

_____

_____

_____

_____

_____

_____

Liquids Log

_____

_____

_____

_____

_____

_____

_____

Sleep
total time _____

Meditation
total time _____

Notes

Date

Exercise Log

_____

_____

_____

_____

_____

_____

_____

_____

_____

_____

_____

_____

Muscles Worked

Total Time _____

Intensity   1   2   3   4   5

Mood   ☹   😐   🙂   😀

Overall   ★ ★ ★ ★ ★

Food Log

_____

_____

_____

_____

_____

_____

_____

Liquids Log

_____

_____

_____

_____

_____

_____

_____

Sleep total time _____

Meditation total time _____

Notes

Date

Exercise Log

_____

_____

_____

_____

_____

_____

_____

_____

_____

_____

_____

_____

Muscles Worked

Total Time

_____

Intensity   1   2   3   4   5

Mood   ☹   😐   🙂   😃

Overall   ★ ★ ★ ★ ★

Food Log

_____

_____

_____

_____

_____

_____

_____

_____

Liquids Log

_____

_____

_____

_____

_____

_____

_____

_____

Sleep
total time _____

Meditation
total time _____

Notes

Date

Exercise Log

_____

_____

_____

_____

_____

_____

_____

_____

_____

_____

Muscles Worked

Total Time _____

Intensity   1   2   3   4   5

Mood   ☹   😐   🙂   😃

Overall   ★ ★ ★ ★ ★

Food Log

_____

_____

_____

_____

_____

_____

_____

Liquids Log

_____

_____

_____

_____

_____

_____

_____

Sleep
total time _____

Meditation
total time _____

Notes

Date _____

Exercise Log

_____

_____

_____

_____

_____

_____

_____

_____

_____

_____

_____

Muscles Worked

Total Time _____

Intensity   1   2   3   4   5

Mood   ☹   😐   🙂   😃

Overall   ★ ★ ★ ★ ★

Food Log

_____

_____

_____

_____

_____

_____

_____

Liquids Log

_____

_____

_____

_____

_____

_____

_____

Sleep
total time _____

Meditation
total time _____

Notes

Date

Exercise Log

_____

_____

_____

_____

_____

_____

_____

_____

_____

_____

_____

_____

Muscles Worked

Total Time _____

Intensity   1   2   3   4   5

Mood   ☹ 😐 🙂 😃

Overall   ★ ★ ★ ★ ★

Food Log

_____

_____

_____

_____

_____

_____

_____

Liquids Log

_____

_____

_____

_____

_____

_____

_____

Sleep
total time _____

Meditation
total time _____

Notes

Date _____

Exercise Log

_____

_____

_____

_____

_____

_____

_____

_____

_____

_____

_____

_____

Muscles Worked

Total Time _____

Intensity   1   2   3   4   5

Mood   :(:| :)   :D

Overall   ★ ★ ★ ★ ★

Food Log

_____

_____

_____

_____

_____

_____

_____

Liquids Log

_____

_____

_____

_____

_____

_____

_____

Sleep
total time _____

Meditation
total time _____

Notes

Date _____

Exercise Log

_____

_____

_____

_____

_____

_____

_____

_____

_____

_____

_____

Muscles Worked

Total Time _____

Intensity   1   2   3   4   5

Mood   ☹   😐   🙂   😃

Overall   ★ ★ ★ ★ ★

Food Log

_____

_____

_____

_____

_____

_____

_____

_____

Liquids Log

_____

_____

_____

_____

_____

_____

_____

_____

Sleep
total time _____

Meditation
total time _____

Notes

Date _____

Exercise Log

_____

_____

_____

_____

_____

_____

_____

_____

_____

_____

_____

_____

Muscles Worked

Total Time _____

Intensity   1   2   3   4   5

Mood   ☹   😐   🙂   😃

Overall   ★ ★ ★ ★ ★

Food Log

_____

_____

_____

_____

_____

_____

_____

Liquids Log

_____

_____

_____

_____

_____

_____

_____

Sleep
total time _____

Meditation
total time _____

Notes

Date _____

Exercise Log

_____

_____

_____

_____

_____

_____

_____

_____

_____

_____

_____

_____

_____

Muscles Worked

Total Time _____

Intensity   1   2   3   4   5

Mood   ☹   😐   🙂   😃

Overall   ⭐ ⭐ ⭐ ⭐ ⭐

Food Log

_____

_____

_____

_____

_____

_____

_____

_____

Liquids Log

_____

_____

_____

_____

_____

_____

_____

_____

Sleep
total time _____

Meditation
total time _____

Notes

Date _____

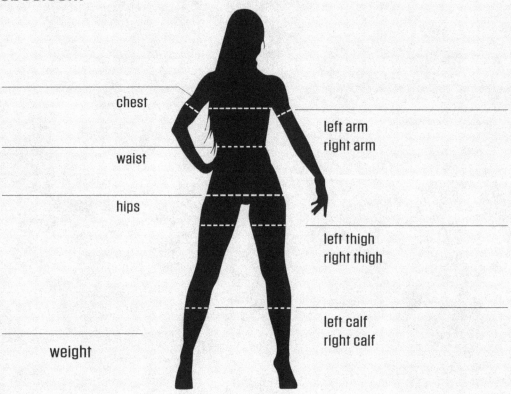

chest

waist

hips

weight

left arm
right arm

left thigh
right thigh

left calf
right calf

Date _____

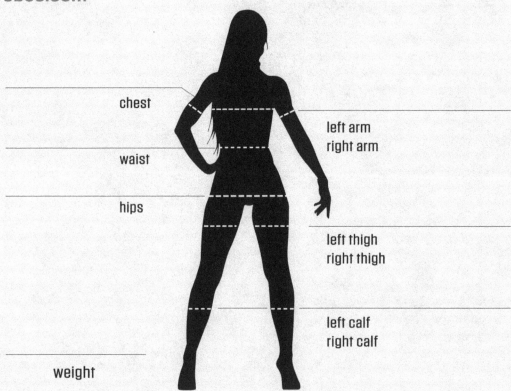

chest

waist

hips

weight

left arm
right arm

left thigh
right thigh

left calf
right calf

Date _____

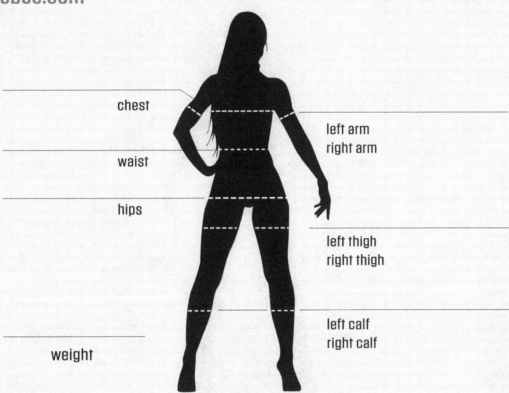

chest

left arm
right arm

waist

hips

left thigh
right thigh

left calf
right calf

weight

Date _____

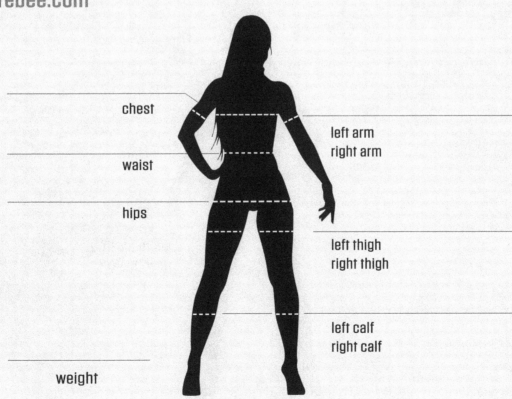

chest

left arm
right arm

waist

hips

left thigh
right thigh

left calf
right calf

weight

Date _____

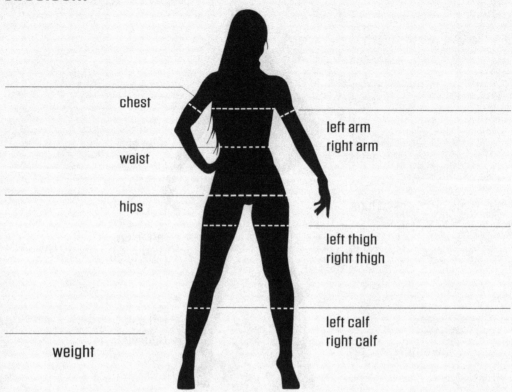

chest

left arm
right arm

waist

hips

left thigh
right thigh

left calf
right calf

weight

Date _____

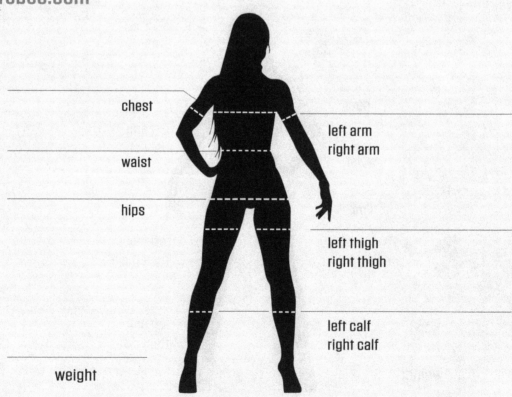

chest

left arm
right arm

waist

hips

left thigh
right thigh

left calf
right calf

weight

Date _____

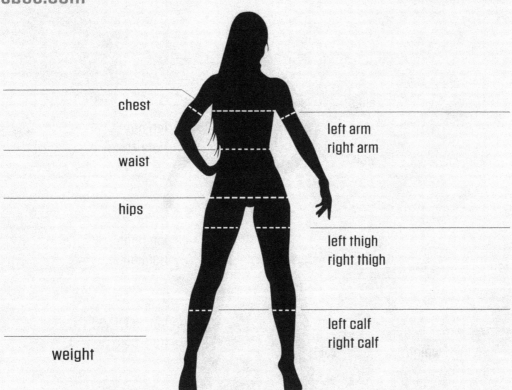

chest

left arm
right arm

waist

hips

left thigh
right thigh

left calf
right calf

_____
weight

Date _____

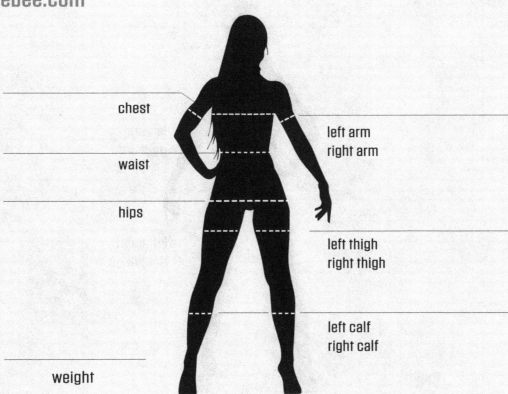

chest

left arm
right arm

waist

hips

left thigh
right thigh

left calf
right calf

_____
weight

Date _____

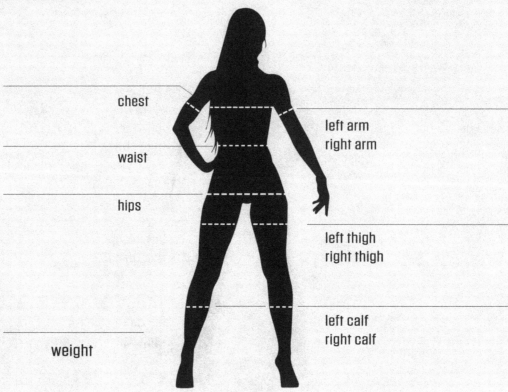

chest

left arm
right arm

waist

hips

left thigh
right thigh

left calf
right calf

weight

Date _____

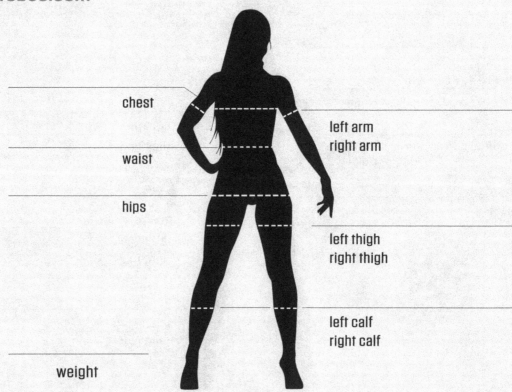

chest

left arm
right arm

waist

hips

left thigh
right thigh

left calf
right calf

weight

Date _____

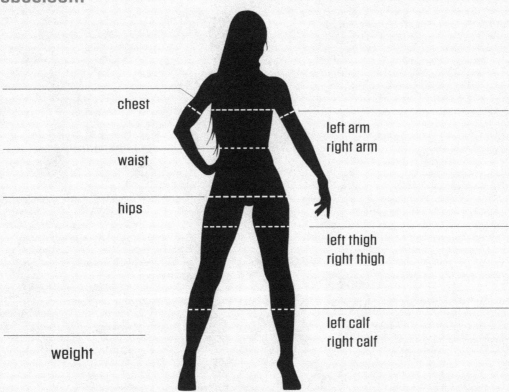

chest

left arm
right arm

waist

hips

left thigh
right thigh

left calf
right calf

weight

Date _____

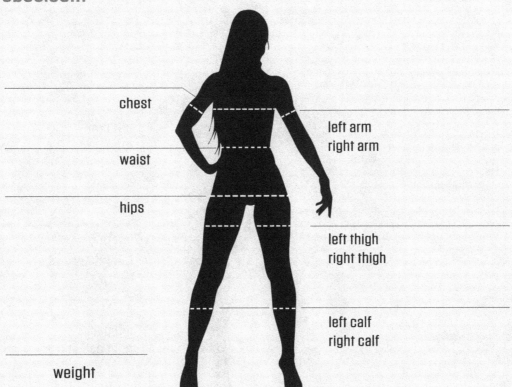

chest

left arm
right arm

waist

hips

left thigh
right thigh

left calf
right calf

weight

Date _____

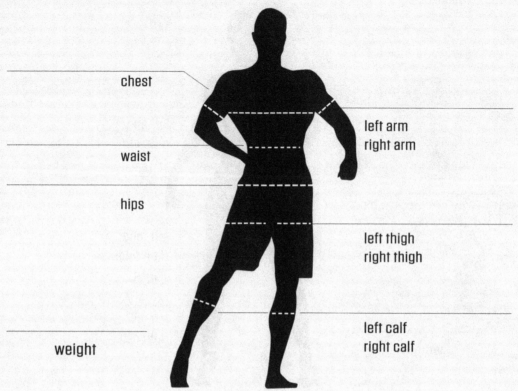

chest

waist

hips

weight

left arm
right arm

left thigh
right thigh

left calf
right calf

Date _____

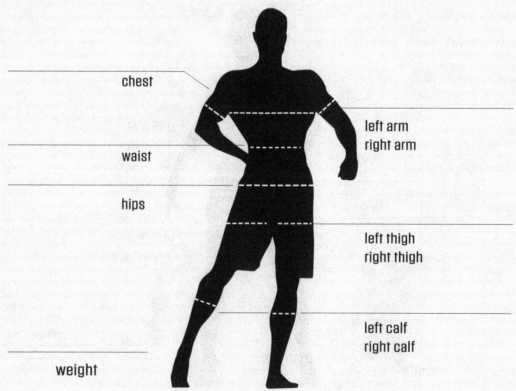

chest

waist

hips

weight

left arm
right arm

left thigh
right thigh

left calf
right calf

Date _____

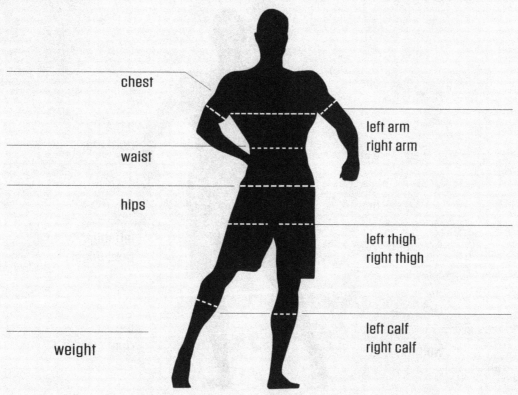

chest

left arm
right arm

waist

hips

left thigh
right thigh

left calf
right calf

weight

Date _____

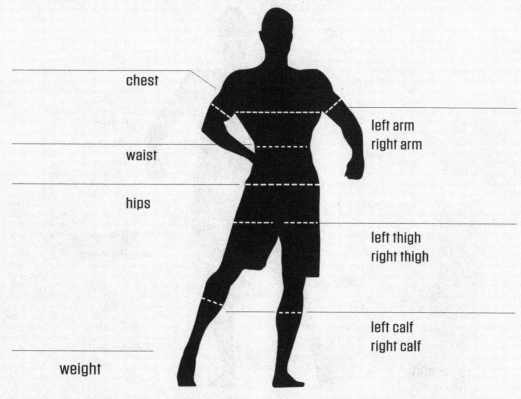

chest

left arm
right arm

waist

hips

left thigh
right thigh

left calf
right calf

weight

Date _____

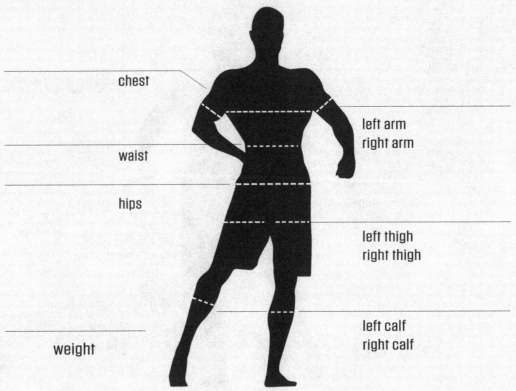

chest

left arm
right arm

waist

hips

left thigh
right thigh

left calf
right calf

weight

Date _____

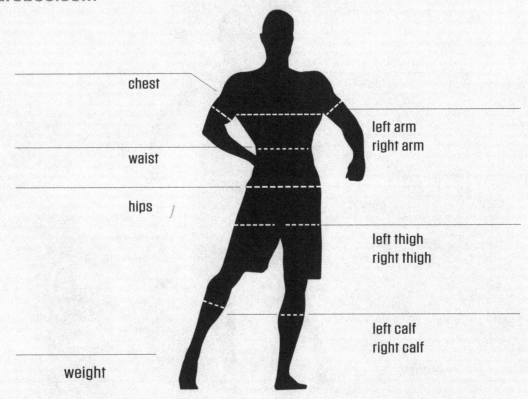

chest

left arm
right arm

waist

hips

left thigh
right thigh

left calf
right calf

weight

Date _____

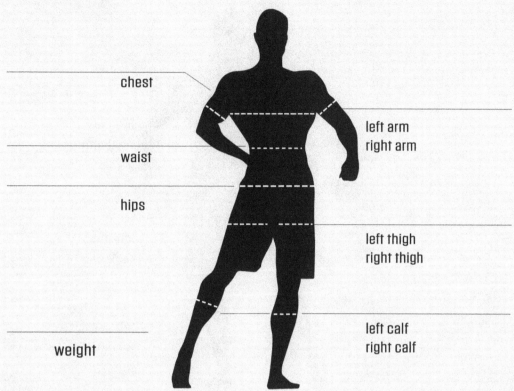

chest

left arm
right arm

waist

hips

left thigh
right thigh

left calf
right calf

weight

Date _____

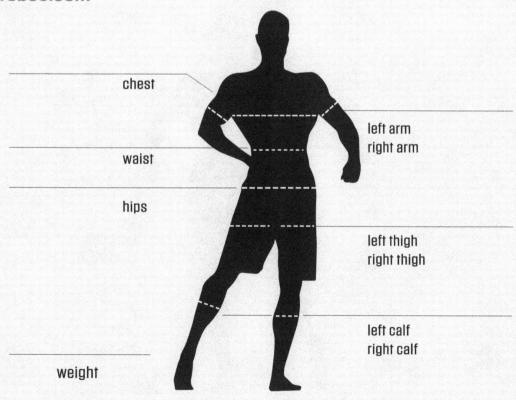

chest

left arm
right arm

waist

hips

left thigh
right thigh

left calf
right calf

weight

Date _____

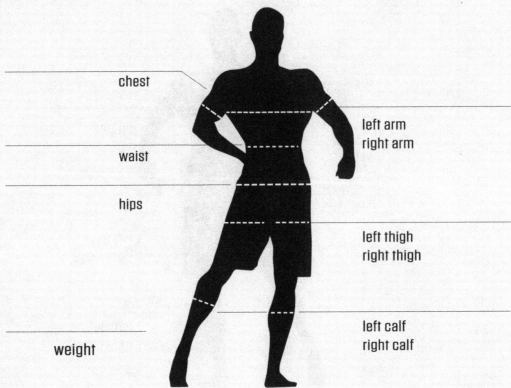

chest

left arm
right arm

waist

hips

left thigh
right thigh

left calf
right calf

weight

Date _____

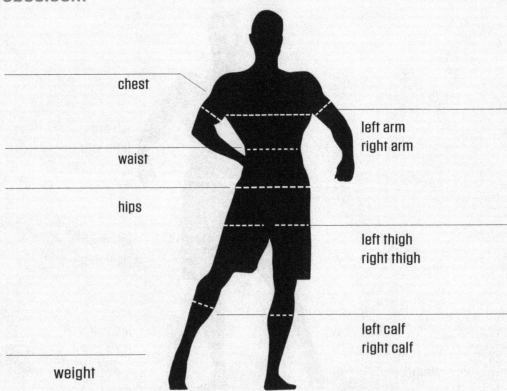

chest

left arm
right arm

waist

hips

left thigh
right thigh

left calf
right calf

weight

Date _____

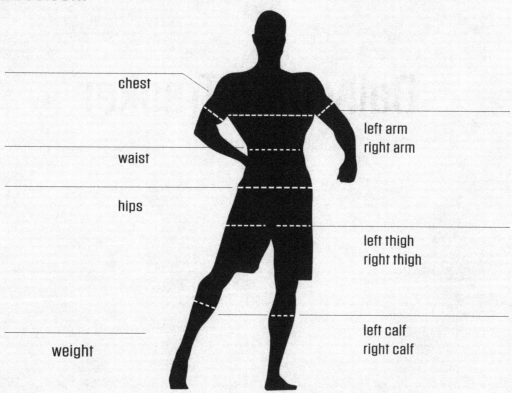

chest

left arm
right arm

waist

hips

left thigh
right thigh

left calf
right calf

weight

Date _____

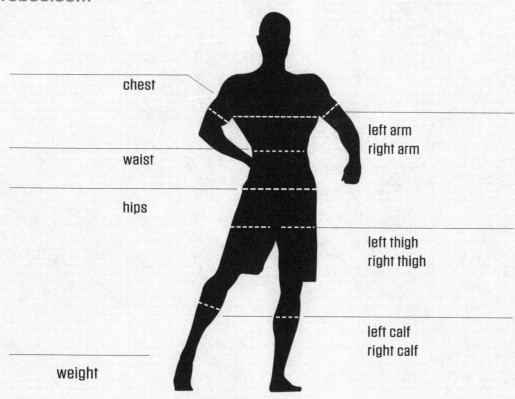

chest

left arm
right arm

waist

hips

left thigh
right thigh

left calf
right calf

weight

Daily Dare Tracker

1	2	3	4	5	6	7	8	9	10
11	12	13	14	15	16	17	18	19	20
21	22	23	24	25	26	27	28	29	30
31	32	33	34	35	36	37	38	39	40
41	42	43	44	45	46	47	48	49	50
51	52	53	54	55	56	57	58	59	60
61	62	63	64	65	66	67	68	69	70
71	72	73	74	75	76	77	78	79	80
81	82	83	84	85	86	87	88	89	90
91	92	93	94	95	96	97	98	99	100

Daily Dares With Extra Credit

© darebee.com

1	2	3	4	5	6	7	8	9	10
11	12	13	14	15	16	17	18	19	20
21	22	23	24	25	26	27	28	29	30
31	32	33	34	35	36	37	38	39	40
41	42	43	44	45	46	47	48	49	50
51	52	53	54	55	56	57	58	59	60
61	62	63	64	65	66	67	68	69	70
71	72	73	74	75	76	77	78	79	80
81	82	83	84	85	86	87	88	89	90
91	92	93	94	95	96	97	98	99	100

Thank you!

Thank you for purchasing 100 No-Equipment Workouts Vol. 3, DAREBEE project print edition. DAREBEE is a non-profit global fitness resource dedicated to making fitness accessible for everyone, no matter their circumstances. The project is supported exclusively via user donations and paperback royalties.

After printing costs and store fees every book developed by the DAREBEE project makes $1 and it goes directly into our project maintenance and development fund.

Each sale helps us keep the DAREBEE resource growing, maintain it and keep it up. Thank you for making a difference in its future!

Other books in this series include:

100 No-Equipment Workouts Vol 1.
100 No-Equipment Workouts Vol 2.
100 No-Equipment Workouts Vol 3.
100 No-Equipment Workouts Vol 4.
100 Office Workouts
Pocket Workouts: 100 no-equipment workouts
ABS 100 Workouts: Visual Easy-To-Follow ABS Exercise Routines for All Fitness Levels
100 HIIT Workouts: Visual easy-to-follow routines for all fitness levels